This book was compiled by Daniel Melehi with the A.I assistance of Inventabot

<u>Dedication</u>

I hope this helps all of my wonderful readers achieve all their goals in their business. And I would like to thank my wonderful wife for all of her continued support in all my ventures.

©Daniel Melehi

May 7 2023

Contents

Introduction

Welcome to "Hidden Health Conditions: Understanding and Treating Lesser-Known Ailments". This book explores a range of health conditions that are not commonly discussed but can have a significant impact on a person's quality of life. It is essential to understand these lesser-known ailments because they can be misdiagnosed or go undiagnosed for years. Many people needlessly suffer because their condition isn't recognized, so the goal of this book is to raise awareness of these conditions and provide information on how individuals can manage their symptoms.

WHY HIDDEN HEALTH CONDITIONS MATTER

Hidden health conditions affect a large number of people, but they often remain undiagnosed and misunderstood for years. These conditions can significantly impact an individual's mental and physical health, their ability to work and study, and their personal relationships. However, because people with hidden health conditions don't always "look sick", their struggles can go unnoticed, leading to feelings of isolation and frustration.

THE IMPORTANCE OF UNDERSTANDING LESSER-KNOWN AILMENTS

By understanding and recognizing hidden health conditions, we can work towards earlier diagnoses and effective treatments. This may involve educating medical professionals and bringing attention to these conditions in public awareness campaigns. It's also essential for those who suffer from these conditions to educate themselves on their symptoms, management, and treatment options.

OVERVIEW OF THE BOOK'S STRUCTURE

The book is divided into seven chapters, each focused on a different area of the body and the corresponding hidden health conditions. Chapter 2 explores hidden digestive system diseases such as Celiac Disease, Gastroparesis, SIBO and Irritable Bowel Syndrome. Chapter 3 dives into the nervous system illnesses which include Fibromyalgia, Chronic Fatigue Syndrome, Restless Leg Syndrome, and Migraines. Chapter 4 discusses auto-immune diseases such as Lupus, Multiple Sclerosis (MS), Sjogren's Syndrome, and Rheumatoid Arthritis (RA). Chapter 5 uncovers the lesser-known ailments that affect other parts of the body including Polycystic Ovary Syndrome (PCOS), Endometriosis, Chronic Lyme Disease, and Meniere's Disease. Chapter 6 examines various treatment options for hidden health conditions, including traditional medical treatments, alternative and complementary therapies, and lifestyle changes. Chapter 7 concludes the book with a recap of the hidden health conditions, a call to action for improved recognition and treatment, and final thoughts and resources. Throughout the book, we hope to provide you with helpful information that expands your knowledge of lesser-known ailments and provides actionable steps to manage the symptoms of these conditions.

WHY HIDDEN HEALTH CONDITIONS MATTER

Hidden health conditions often go unnoticed, misdiagnosed, or mistreated. These conditions are difficult to diagnose and treat because they are not as common as other well-known diseases. Even healthcare providers may not recognize the symptoms or have the necessary knowledge to diagnose and treat them. As a result, patients may suffer for years, seeing multiple specialists, undergoing various tests, and taking ineffective treatments. Hidden health conditions may include autoimmune disorders, digestive disorders, neurological disorders, and hormonal imbalances, among others. They can cause chronic pain, fatigue, cognitive impairment, digestive distress, skin problems, and other symptoms that affect the quality of life. Moreover, hidden health conditions can be stigmatized because they are not well-understood or widely recognized. Patients may face skepticism, indifference, or dismissiveness from others, including friends, family members, coworkers, and even healthcare providers. This can lead to social isolation, depression, anxiety, and reduced productivity. Therefore, it is essential to raise awareness about hidden health conditions, both among the general public and healthcare professionals. By doing so, we can increase the chances of early diagnosis and effective treatment, reduce the burden of suffering, and improve the lives of millions of people living with hidden health conditions. In the following subchapters, we will discuss some of the most common hidden health conditions, their symptoms, causes, diagnoses, and treatments. We will also provide tips on how to manage these conditions and improve your overall health and well-being.

CHAPTER 1: INTRODUCTION

Subchapter 1.2: The Importance of Understanding Lesser-Known Ailments

As important as it is to remain aware of the common health conditions that people face, it is equally critical to understand less well-known ailments that can be equally debilitating and life-altering. There are countless health conditions that receive significantly less attention than others, as well as countless individuals who quietly suffer from them. The lack of awareness and attention to these health conditions means that people who have them may go undiagnosed or undertreated, which can lead to worsening health outcomes and make it even more difficult for these individuals to live a full and healthy life. Many of these lesser-known ailments still require medical treatment and intervention, but they might require a more nuanced approach than the more widely recognized conditions. For example, many autoimmune conditions are difficult to diagnose, and they can present a range of symptoms that are not immediately obvious as being connected to a larger health condition. Without a proper diagnosis, people with autoimmune conditions may go years without proper treatment, developing significant health problems as a result. The importance of understanding lesser-known ailments can't be emphasized enough. Even if they are less prevalent in our society, they still require attention from healthcare professionals, policymakers, and the general public. By putting a spotlight on these conditions and raising awareness of them, we can help ensure that people living with them can get the support and care they need.

In the following chapters, we will explore a range of lesser-known ailments that people face, offering insight into their causes, effects, and potential treatments. With each chapter, our goal is not only to inform readers of these conditions but to empower them with the tools they need to recognize the signs and symptoms of these conditions and take action to get the help they need.

OVERVIEW OF THE BOOK'S STRUCTURE

This book, Hidden Health Conditions: Understanding and Treating Lesser-Known Ailments, is designed to be a comprehensive guide to a diverse range of health conditions that are often misunderstood or misdiagnosed. The book is divided into seven chapters, each focused on a different aspect of hidden health conditions. Chapter 1 provides an introduction to the importance of understanding these conditions and how this book is structured to help readers gain a better understanding of the various ailments. Chapters 2 to 4 focus on specific systems of the body, including the digestive, nervous, and immune systems. Within each chapter, we cover several lesser-known conditions that often go undiagnosed, misdiagnosed, or ignored by medical professionals. Some of the conditions covered include celiac disease, gastroparesis, fibromyalgia, multiple sclerosis, and lupus. Chapter 5 is a catch-all for other lesser-known ailments that don't fit neatly into a specific system, such as PCOS, endometriosis, chronic Lyme disease, and Meniere's disease. Chapter 6 covers various treatment options for hidden health conditions, including traditional medical treatments, alternative and complementary therapies, and lifestyle changes for long-term management. Finally, Chapter 7 provides a recap of the book's contents, a call to action for better recognition and treatment of these conditions, and additional resources for readers seeking additional information. Overall, this book aims to provide readers with a comprehensive and informative resource on lesser-known health conditions, including tips and strategies for managing them effectively.

Chapter 2: The Digestive System

The digestive system is responsible for breaking down food and absorbing nutrients. However, there are some hidden health conditions that can cause problems for the digestive system. This chapter will explore some of these conditions and provide an overview of their symptoms and treatment options.

SUBCHAPTER 2.1: CELIAC DISEASE

Celiac disease is an autoimmune disorder that affects the small intestine. People with celiac disease are unable to tolerate gluten, a protein found in wheat, rye, and barley. When someone with celiac disease eats gluten, their immune system attacks their small intestine, causing damage and preventing the absorption of essential nutrients. Symptoms of celiac disease include bloating, diarrhea, constipation, abdominal pain, and weight loss. Treatment for celiac disease involves following a strict gluten-free diet. This means avoiding all foods that contain wheat, rye, and barley. People with celiac disease should also avoid foods that may be cross-contaminated with gluten, such as those prepared with the same equipment as gluten-containing foods.

SUBCHAPTER 2.2: GASTROPARESIS

Gastroparesis is a condition that affects the normal movement of food through the stomach. It occurs when the muscles in the stomach are weak or damaged, preventing food from being properly digested and moving through the digestive tract. The most common symptoms of gastroparesis include nausea, vomiting, bloating, and abdominal pain. Treatment options for gastroparesis include medication therapy and changes to the diet. In some cases, a feeding tube may be necessary to ensure the patient is getting adequate nutrition.

SUBCHAPTER 2.3: SMALL INTESTINAL BACTERIAL OVERGROWTH (SIBO)

Small intestinal bacterial overgrowth (SIBO) is a condition where there is too much bacteria in the small intestine. This can cause a variety of symptoms, including bloating, diarrhea, constipation, and abdominal pain. SIBO can be caused by a number of factors, including gut dysbiosis, autoimmune disorders, and poor diet. Treatment for SIBO often involves a combination of dietary changes and antibiotic therapy. Patients may also be advised to take probiotics to help maintain a healthy balance of bacteria in the gut.

SUBCHAPTER 2.4: IRRITABLE BOWEL SYNDROME (IBS)

Irritable bowel syndrome (IBS) is a chronic condition that affects the large intestine. It is characterized by a group of symptoms, including abdominal pain, bloating, constipation, and diarrhea. The exact cause of IBS is unknown, but it is thought to be related to changes in the gut microbiome and increased sensitivity in the intestines. Treatment for IBS may involve changes to the diet, stress reduction techniques, and medication therapy. In some cases, a low-FODMAP diet may be recommended to help manage symptoms. In conclusion, there are several hidden health conditions that can affect the digestive system. It is important to recognize the symptoms of these conditions and seek proper medical treatment. If you are experiencing any digestive issues, be sure to talk to your healthcare provider to determine the underlying cause and explore treatment options.

SUBCHAPTER 2.1: CELIAC DISEASE

Celiac disease is an autoimmune disorder that affects roughly 1 in 100 people worldwide. This condition results when gluten, a protein found in wheat, barley, and rye, triggers an immune response in the body. Over time, this immune reaction damages the small intestine and interferes with nutrient absorption. Symptoms of celiac disease can vary widely from person to person. Some individuals may experience gastrointestinal symptoms such as bloating, diarrhea, abdominal pain, and nausea. Others may experience non-digestive symptoms such as anemia, fatigue, headache, joint pain, and skin rash. In some cases, people with celiac disease may have no symptoms at all. Diagnosing celiac disease involves a combination of blood tests and biopsies of the small intestine. A blood test can screen for autoantibodies that are commonly present with celiac disease. If the blood test is positive, a biopsy of the small intestine can confirm the diagnosis. The treatment for celiac disease is a lifelong gluten-free diet. This means avoiding all foods that contain wheat, barley, and rye. For some individuals, a gluten-free diet can bring about improvement in symptoms within weeks. However, it can take up to two years for the intestine to heal completely. It is important to note that gluten is not harmful to most people. For people with celiac disease, however, consuming gluten can cause serious health consequences in the long term. Therefore, it is crucial for those with celiac disease to maintain a strict gluten-free diet. In addition to dietary changes, people with celiac disease may also benefit from seeing a registered dietitian or physician who specializes in celiac disease management. These experts can help ensure that a gluten-free diet is nutritionally balanced and provide guidance on how to manage the condition effectively. If left untreated, celiac disease can lead to a variety of complications including malnutrition, osteoporosis, infertility, and even cancer. Therefore, it is important to seek diagnosis and treatment as soon as possible if celiac disease is suspected.

SUBCHAPTER 2.2: GASTROPARESIS

Gastroparesis is a condition in which the stomach muscles cannot properly contract to move food through the digestive tract. This can cause food to stay in the stomach for an extended period of time, leading to uncomfortable symptoms such as nausea, vomiting, and abdominal pain. The exact cause of gastroparesis is often unknown, but it can be associated with diabetes, certain medications, Parkinson's disease, and other nervous system disorders. It can also develop after surgery or as a result of an infection. Symptoms of gastroparesis may include feeling full after only a few bites of food, heartburn, bloating, and decreased appetite. Diagnosing gastroparesis can involve tests such as gastric emptying studies, upper endoscopy, and imaging studies. Treatment options for gastroparesis often aim to manage symptoms and promote proper digestion. This may include dietary changes such as consuming smaller and more frequent meals, avoiding high-fat and high-fiber foods, and drinking plenty of fluids. Medications such as prokinetic agents and antiemetics may also be prescribed to help promote gastric motility and reduce nausea and vomiting. In severe cases of gastroparesis, more invasive treatments such as feeding tubes or surgery may be recommended. It is important to work closely with a healthcare team to determine the most appropriate treatment plan for individual cases of gastroparesis.

SUBCHAPTER 2.3: SMALL INTESTINAL BACTERIAL OVERGROWTH (SIBO)

Small Intestinal Bacterial Overgrowth, commonly known as SIBO, is a condition where there are too many bacteria in the small intestine. The small intestine is the part of the digestive system where the majority of nutrients are absorbed into the body. In a healthy person, there are relatively low levels of bacteria in the small intestine, but in those with SIBO, there are too many bacteria, which can lead to a range of symptoms. These symptoms can include bloating, gas, abdominal pain, diarrhea, and constipation. SIBO can also lead to malabsorption of nutrients, which can result in deficiencies in vitamins and other essential nutrients. One of the main causes of SIBO is a problem with the structure or function of the digestive system. For example, a person with a structural issue, such as a bowel obstruction or narrowing, may be more susceptible to SIBO. Similarly, those with digestive system motility issues, such as people with diabetes or scleroderma, may also be more prone to SIBO. The treatment for SIBO involves reducing the number of bacteria in the small intestine and treating any underlying conditions that may be contributing to the problem. Antibiotics are often used to reduce the bacteria, but dietary changes can also be effective. A low-FODMAP diet, which restricts certain types of carbohydrates that are commonly fermented by gut bacteria, has been shown to be effective in managing symptoms of SIBO. However, it's important to note that SIBO can be a chronic condition, and managing symptoms may require ongoing treatment and lifestyle modifications. Consulting with a healthcare professional is essential for proper diagnosis and treatment. In summary, SIBO is a condition where there are too many bacteria in the small intestine, leading to a variety of digestive symptoms and nutrient malabsorption. Treatment typically involves reducing the bacteria through antibiotics or dietary changes, but ongoing management may be necessary. If you suspect you may have SIBO, it's important to speak with a healthcare professional to receive proper diagnosis and treatment.

SUBCHAPTER 2.4: IRRITABLE BOWEL SYNDROME (IBS)

IBS is a gastrointestinal disorder that affects the large intestine. Symptoms may include abdominal pain, bloating, constipation or diarrhea, and gas. IBS affects approximately 10-15% of the population and is twice as common in women as in men. Although the exact cause of IBS is not known, it is believed to be related to food sensitivity, stress, bacterial overgrowth, or hormonal changes. IBS can be diagnosed through a series of tests that include a physical examination, stool tests, blood tests, and colonoscopy. There is currently no cure for IBS, but its symptoms can be managed through dietary changes, stress management, medication, and probiotics. It is important to work closely with a healthcare provider to create a personalized treatment plan based on the individual's needs. Dietary changes may include eliminating certain foods from the diet, such as dairy products, gluten, fatty foods, and high-fiber foods. Stress management techniques, such as deep breathing, meditation, and regular exercise, can also help alleviate symptoms. Medications that may be used to manage IBS include antispasmodics, which relax the muscles in the intestines, and laxatives, which help with constipation. Probiotics may help rebalance the gut microbiome and reduce symptoms of IBS. In summary, IBS is a common gastrointestinal disorder that requires a personalized approach to treatment. By identifying triggers and working closely with a healthcare provider, individuals with IBS can successfully manage their symptoms and improve their quality of life.

Chapter 3: The Nervous System

The nervous system is responsible for controlling and coordinating all the functions within the body. When this system is not functioning properly, it can lead to a variety of health conditions and ailments. In this chapter, we will explore some of the lesser-known ailments that affect the nervous system and how they can be treated.

SUBCHAPTER 3.1: FIBROMYALGIA

Fibromyalgia is a chronic disorder that affects the muscles and soft tissues. The symptoms of fibromyalgia can include fatigue, pain, and tenderness in various parts of the body, as well as cognitive difficulties. Although there is no known cure for fibromyalgia, there are treatments that can help manage the symptoms. Some of the common treatments for fibromyalgia include medications such as pain relievers, antidepressants, and anticonvulsants. Lifestyle changes such as exercise, stress management, and appropriate sleep hygiene may also help manage the symptoms of fibromyalgia. Alternative therapies such as acupuncture, massage, and cognitive-behavioral therapy have also been shown to be effective in some patients.

SUBCHAPTER 3.2: CHRONIC FATIGUE SYNDROME

Chronic fatigue syndrome (CFS) is a debilitating condition characterized by extreme fatigue that is not relieved by rest. Other symptoms of CFS can include headaches, joint pain, and cognitive difficulties. The cause of CFS is not yet fully understood, but it is believed to be related to dysfunction in the immune system and hypothalamic-pituitary-adrenal (HPA) axis. The treatment for CFS is primarily focused on managing the symptoms. This may include medications such as pain relievers, antidepressants, and sleeping aids. Lifestyle changes such as regular exercise, appropriate sleep hygiene, and stress management can also help manage the symptoms of CFS. Cognitive-behavioral therapy has also been shown to be effective in helping patients improve their quality of life.

SUBCHAPTER 3.3: RESTLESS LEG SYNDROME

Restless leg syndrome (RLS) is a neurological disorder that causes an irresistible urge to move the legs. This sensation is often described as a creeping or crawling feeling in the legs, which can be alleviated by movement. RLS can interfere with sleep and cause disruptions to daily life. The treatment for RLS may include medications such as dopamine agonists, anticonvulsants, and opioids. Lifestyle changes such as regular exercise, avoiding caffeine and alcohol, and establishing a regular sleep routine can also help manage the symptoms of RLS. Iron supplements may also be recommended for patients with low iron levels.

SUBCHAPTER 3.4: MIGRAINES

Migraines are a type of headache that is characterized by intense, throbbing pain on one side of the head. Other symptoms of migraines can include sensitivity to light and sound, nausea, and vomiting. Migraines can be triggered by a variety of factors such as stress, certain foods, and hormonal changes. The treatment for migraines may include medications such as pain relievers, triptans, and anti-nausea medications. Lifestyle changes such as stress management, regular exercise, and avoiding triggers can also help manage the symptoms of migraines. Alternative therapies such as acupuncture and biofeedback have also been shown to be effective in some patients. In conclusion, the nervous system plays a crucial role in regulating bodily functions, and any disruptions to its normal function can lead to various health conditions. Understanding the lesser-known ailments that affect the nervous system and how they can be treated can help patients manage their symptoms and improve their quality of life.

CHAPTER 3: THE NERVOUS SYSTEM

Subchapter 3.1: Fibromyalgia

Fibromyalgia is a chronic disorder characterized by widespread musculoskeletal pain, fatigue, and tenderness in localized areas. It affects approximately 2% to 8% of the population, with women being more commonly affected than men. The exact cause of fibromyalgia is unknown, but researchers believe that multiple factors can contribute to its development, including genetics, infections, physical or emotional trauma, and abnormal pain processing in the central nervous system. The most common symptoms of fibromyalgia are pain, fatigue, and sleep disturbances. The pain can vary in severity and can be described as a dull ache, a shooting or burning pain, or as muscle twitching or soreness. It is typically felt throughout the body and is often accompanied by tenderness in localized areas such as the neck, shoulders, back, hips, and legs. The fatigue experienced by fibromyalgia patients can be so severe that it interferes with daily activities and can be described as a constant feeling of exhaustion. Sleep disturbances are also common in fibromyalgia patients and can include difficulty falling asleep, staying asleep, or waking up feeling unrested. Currently, there is no known cure for fibromyalgia, but there are a variety of treatment options available that can help alleviate its symptoms. Treatment options can include medication, physical therapy, occupational therapy, and counseling. Medications such as pain relievers, antidepressants, and anti-seizure drugs may be prescribed to help manage pain, fatigue, and sleep disturbances. Physical and occupational therapy can also be helpful in managing fibromyalgia symptoms by improving strength, flexibility, and overall mobility. Counseling may also be beneficial for individuals with fibromyalgia, as it can help them manage the emotional and psychological effects of chronic pain and fatigue. Techniques such as cognitive-behavioral therapy and mindfulness-based stress reduction are often effective in managing stress and anxiety associated with chronic pain conditions. In conclusion, fibromyalgia is a chronic disorder that can significantly impact an individual's quality of life. Its symptoms can be physically and emotionally debilitating, but treatment options are available to help manage pain, fatigue, and other associated symptoms. It is important for individuals with fibromyalgia to work closely with their healthcare providers to find a treatment plan that works best for them.

CHAPTER 3: THE NERVOUS SYSTEM

Subchapter 3.2: Chronic Fatigue Syndrome

Chronic fatigue syndrome (CFS), also known as myalgic encephalomyelitis (ME), is a complex and often misunderstood condition. It is characterized by persistent fatigue that is not relieved by rest and is not the result of an underlying medical condition. This fatigue also cannot be explained by any other medical or mental health disorder. People with CFS often experience a range of symptoms, including muscle pain, joint pain, headaches, sleep disturbances, and cognitive difficulties. These symptoms can be severe and can adversely affect a person's quality of life. The causes of CFS are not fully understood, but it is believed to be related to dysfunction in the immune, endocrine, and nervous systems. Factors that may contribute to the development of CFS include viral infections, immune system dysfunction, hormonal imbalances, and stress. Currently, there is no cure for CFS. Treatment focuses on managing symptoms and improving quality of life. This may include a combination of medication, therapy, and lifestyle changes. A multidisciplinary approach that involves healthcare professionals from different disciplines can be helpful in managing and treating CFS. It is important for individuals with CFS to work closely with their healthcare team to develop a customized treatment plan that addresses their unique needs. With the right treatment and support, many people with CFS are able to achieve improved functioning and quality of life.

CHAPTER 3: THE NERVOUS SYSTEM

Subchapter 3.3: Restless Leg Syndrome

Restless Leg Syndrome (RLS) is a nervous system disorder that causes an overwhelming urge to move your legs, especially when you're trying to relax or sleep. This can lead to disruption of your sleep patterns and cause daytime fatigue. RLS affects up to 10% of the population, and the cause is still unknown. However, it can often be linked to family history. RLS can also be a symptom of other underlying conditions such as iron deficiency anemia, peripheral neuropathy, or pregnancy. Common symptoms of RLS include an uncontrollable urge to move your legs, uncomfortable sensations in your legs such as tingling, crawling, itching, or pulling, and worsening of symptoms during periods of inactivity or rest. Treatment of RLS includes medications to increase dopamine levels in the brain, which can help relieve restless leg symptoms. Other medication treatments include opioids, anticonvulsants, and muscle relaxants. Additionally, lifestyle changes such as regular exercise, avoiding caffeine and alcohol, and maintaining a regular sleep schedule can also help manage symptoms. In severe cases, RLS can interfere with your quality of life, but with the right treatment, most people with RLS can lead a happy and healthy life. If you believe you may have RLS, it is important to talk to your healthcare provider about your symptoms and potential treatment options. Overall, RLS is a lesser-known ailment that affects many people. By understanding the symptoms and seeking the right treatment, individuals with RLS can improve their quality of life.

CHAPTER 3: THE NERVOUS SYSTEM

Subchapter 3.4: Migraines

Migraines are a type of headache that is often recurring and can be debilitating. They affect millions of people worldwide and are more common in women than in men. A migraine can cause severe pain, sensitivity to light and sound, and nausea. Migraines are different from a normal headache because they come with other symptoms like visual disturbances, and tingling in the fingers. The headache usually starts on one side of the head and is characterized by a throbbing or pulsing sensation. There are various triggers of migraines, including hormonal changes, stress, certain foods, or changes in weather. It's essential to be aware of your triggers so that you can avoid them if possible. Treatment for migraines can include pain medication, lifestyle changes, and alternative therapies like massage and acupuncture. Prevention is crucial in managing migraines, so it's essential to learn about your triggers, manage your stress levels, and maintain consistent sleep patterns. If you are experiencing migraines, it's crucial to talk to your healthcare provider to develop a treatment plan that is best for you. Migraines can be managed, and with the right plan in place, they do not have to control your life.

Chapter 4: The Immune System

The immune system is the body's defense mechanism against foreign invaders such as bacteria and viruses. However, sometimes the immune system can turn against the body itself, leading to autoimmune diseases. In this chapter, we will explore some of the lesser-known autoimmune diseases that can seriously impact a person's health and quality of life.

SUBCHAPTER 4.1: LUPUS

Lupus, also known as systemic lupus erythematosus (SLE), is a chronic autoimmune disease in which the immune system attacks healthy tissues and organs, such as the skin, joints, kidneys, brain, and heart. This can cause inflammation, pain, and damage to these organs. Lupus can be difficult to diagnose as it shares symptoms with many other conditions, but common symptoms include fatigue, joint pain, skin rashes, and fever. Treatment options may include anti-inflammatory medications, corticosteroids, immunosuppressants, and lifestyle changes such as avoiding sun exposure.

SUBCHAPTER 4.2: MULTIPLE SCLEROSIS (MS)

Multiple sclerosis, or MS, is a chronic autoimmune disease that affects the central nervous system, including the brain and spinal cord. MS occurs when the immune system attacks and damages the protective myelin coating around nerve fibers, leading to communication issues between the brain and the rest of the body. Symptoms of MS can vary greatly but may include muscle weakness, difficulty with coordination and balance, visual disturbances, and cognitive problems. Treatment may include disease-modifying therapies, medications to manage symptoms, physical therapy, and lifestyle changes to promote general health.

SUBCHAPTER 4.3: SJOGREN'S SYNDROME

Sjogren's syndrome is an autoimmune disease that primarily affects the glands that produce moisture, such as the salivary and tear glands. This can lead to dry and irritated eyes, mouth, and throat, as well as other complications such as joint pain and dry skin. Sjogren's syndrome can also affect other parts of the body, such as the kidneys, liver, and lungs. There is no cure for

Sjogren's syndrome, but treatment may include medications to manage symptoms, lifestyle changes, and in some cases, immunosuppressive therapy.

SUBCHAPTER 4.4: RHEUMATOID ARTHRITIS (RA)

Rheumatoid arthritis, or RA, is a chronic autoimmune disease that affects the joints of the body, causing inflammation and pain. RA occurs when the immune system attacks the lining of the joints, leading to damage, swelling, and stiffness. RA can also affect other systems of the body, including the skin, eyes, lungs, and blood vessels. Symptoms of RA may include joint pain and stiffness, fatigue, and a general feeling of sickness. Treatment options may include medications such as nonsteroidal anti-inflammatory drugs (NSAIDs), disease-modifying antirheumatic drugs (DMARDs), and biologic response modifiers (biologics). Lifestyle changes, such as regular exercise and maintaining a healthy weight, can also be beneficial.

Conclusion

Autoimmune diseases of the immune system can have a significant impact on a person's health and well-being. Proper diagnosis and management are crucial for those affected by these conditions. If you or a loved one experiences symptoms that may be related to autoimmune disease, it is important to seek medical attention and explore potential treatment options.

CHAPTER 4: THE IMMUNE SYSTEM

Subchapter 4.1: Lupus

Lupus, also called systemic lupus erythematosus or SLE, is a chronic autoimmune disease that can affect many different parts of the body. It occurs when the immune system attacks the body's own tissues and organs, mistaking them for foreign invaders like bacteria or viruses. Symptoms of lupus can vary widely depending on which parts of the body are affected, but some common symptoms include: - Fatigue - Joint pain and swelling - Skin rashes, particularly on the face and neck - Sensitivity to sunlight - Fever - Headaches - Raynaud's phenomenon (where fingers and toes turn white or blue in response to cold or stress) - Shortness of breath Lupus is a complex disease and can be difficult to diagnose because symptoms can mimic those of other illnesses. Medical history, physical exams, blood tests, and imaging tests are often used to help diagnose lupus. While there is no cure for lupus, treatment options are available to manage symptoms and prevent organ damage. Medications such as corticosteroids, immunosuppressants, and antimalarials can help reduce inflammation and prevent the immune system from attacking healthy tissues. Lifestyle changes such as getting enough rest, protecting skin from the sun, and staying physically active can also help manage symptoms. It's important for people with lupus to work closely with their healthcare team to monitor their symptoms and adjust treatment plans as needed. With the right care, many people with lupus are able to manage their symptoms and live full, active lives.

CHAPTER 4: THE IMMUNE SYSTEM

Subchapter 4.2: Multiple Sclerosis (MS)

Multiple sclerosis, commonly referred to as MS, is a chronic autoimmune disease that affects the central nervous system (CNS). In MS, the immune system attacks the myelin sheath that surrounds and protects nerve fibers, causing inflammation and damage to the CNS. MS can cause a wide range of symptoms, including numbness or tingling in the limbs, muscle weakness, difficulty with coordination and balance, blurred or double vision, and cognitive impairment. Symptoms may come and go, making it difficult to diagnose and treat. Currently, there is no cure for MS, but there are treatments available that can help manage symptoms and slow the progression of the disease. Medications such as beta-interferons and glatiramer acetate can reduce the frequency and severity of relapses. Other medications such as dimethyl fumarate, teriflunomide, and fingolimod can also help to reduce inflammation and prevent relapses. In addition to medication, physical therapy and occupational therapy can be helpful in managing MS symptoms. Physical therapy can help with balance, strength, and mobility, while occupational therapy can help with daily activities and maintaining independence. Making lifestyle changes such as exercise, a healthy diet, and stress management can also be beneficial in managing MS. Additionally, alternative therapies such as acupuncture, massage therapy, and yoga may provide some relief for MS symptoms. It's important for people with MS to work closely with their healthcare team to develop a comprehensive treatment plan that takes into account their individual needs and symptoms. With the right treatment and support, people with MS can lead full and active lives.

Conclusion

MS can be a challenging condition to manage, but with the right treatment and lifestyle changes, it's possible to manage symptoms and maintain quality of life. If you or a loved one has been diagnosed with MS, it's important to work closely with healthcare professionals to develop a treatment plan that is tailored to your individual needs. Remember, there is hope and support available for those living with MS.

CHAPTER 4: THE IMMUNE SYSTEM

Subchapter 4.3: Sjogren's Syndrome

Sjogren's Syndrome is an autoimmune disorder affecting approximately 4 million Americans, mostly women over the age of 40. It is a chronic condition where the immune system attacks the exocrine glands, mainly the salivary and lacrimal glands, resulting in dry mouth and dry eyes. In addition to dryness of the mouth and eyes, individuals with Sjogren's Syndrome may also experience joint pain, skin rashes, chronic fatigue, and difficulty swallowing. The severity of the symptoms can vary greatly, and some individuals may also develop other autoimmune disorders such as lupus or rheumatoid arthritis. Diagnosis of Sjogren's Syndrome is often tricky as its symptoms are similar to other autoimmune disorders. However, diagnostic tests such as the Schirmer's test (to measure tear production), the Rose Bengal test (to detect corneal and conjunctival epithelial damage), and blood tests to measure antibodies and inflammation levels, can help to identify the syndrome. There is no known cure for Sjogren's Syndrome, but various treatment options are available to alleviate symptoms and improve quality of life. Artificial tears, ocular lubricants, and saliva substitutes can help to treat dryness. Nonsteroidal anti-inflammatory drugs (NSAIDs) and disease-modifying anti-rheumatic drugs (DMARDs) may also be prescribed to control joint pain and inflammation. Lifestyle changes such as staying hydrated, avoiding irritants, and taking frequent breaks while reading or using electronic devices can all help to manage symptoms. In severe cases, surgery may be recommended to help restore moisture to the eyes and mouth. In conclusion, Sjogren's Syndrome is a chronic autoimmune disorder that affects millions of people worldwide. While there is no known cure, treatment options are available to manage symptoms and improve quality of life. Early diagnosis and management of the symptoms can significantly improve outcomes for individuals with this disorder.

RHEUMATOID ARTHRITIS (RA)

Rheumatoid arthritis is a chronic autoimmune disorder that primarily affects the joints. The disease occurs when the immune system mistakenly attacks the body's own tissues, causing inflammation and, over time, joint damage.

Symptoms

Symptoms of rheumatoid arthritis can vary widely from person to person. Some of the most common symptoms include swollen and painful joints, stiffness, fatigue, and fever. Symptoms may come and go, with periods of active disease (flare-ups) alternating with periods of remission. In severe cases, rheumatoid arthritis can also affect other parts of the body, including the eyes, lungs, and blood vessels.

Causes and Risk Factors

The exact cause of rheumatoid arthritis is unknown, but researchers believe that it may be caused by a combination of genetic and environmental factors. Certain lifestyle factors, such as smoking and obesity, may also increase a person's risk of developing rheumatoid arthritis. Women are also more likely to develop the disease than men.

Treatment Options

There is no cure for rheumatoid arthritis, but a variety of treatment options are available to help manage symptoms and slow the progression of joint damage. These may include medications, such as nonsteroidal anti-inflammatory drugs (NSAIDs) and disease-modifying antirheumatic drugs (DMARDs), as well as physical therapy and lifestyle changes. In cases where joint damage is severe, surgery may be necessary.

Alternative and Complementary Therapies

Many people with rheumatoid arthritis also turn to complementary and alternative therapies to help manage symptoms. Some of these may include acupuncture, massage, yoga, and dietary supplements. While these therapies may provide some relief for some people, it is important to talk to a healthcare professional before trying any new treatments.

Lifestyle Changes

Making certain lifestyle changes can also help manage symptoms of rheumatoid arthritis and improve quality of life. This may include getting regular exercise, maintaining a healthy weight, eating a balanced diet, and getting enough rest and sleep. If you suspect that you may have rheumatoid arthritis, it is important to talk to a healthcare professional for a proper diagnosis and treatment plan. With the right management, many people with rheumatoid arthritis are able to lead active, fulfilling lives.

Chapter 5: Other Lesser-Known Ailments

When it comes to health conditions, there are some that are more well-known than others. In this chapter, we will explore some of the lesser-known ailments that can have a significant impact on a person's quality of life.

SUBCHAPTER 5.1: POLYCYSTIC OVARY SYNDROME (PCOS)

Polycystic Ovary Syndrome (PCOS) is a hormonal disorder that affects women of reproductive age. Women with PCOS may experience irregular periods, difficulty getting pregnant, and other symptoms such as acne and excess hair growth. PCOS is a common condition, affecting up to 1 in 10 women. While the exact cause of PCOS is unknown, it is thought to be related to insulin resistance and elevated levels of male hormones (androgens). Treatment options for PCOS may include lifestyle changes, such as exercise and weight loss, as well as medication to regulate menstrual cycles and hormone levels.

SUBCHAPTER 5.2: ENDOMETRIOSIS

Endometriosis is a painful condition in which tissue similar to the lining of the uterus grows outside of the uterus. This tissue can grow on the ovaries, Fallopian tubes, and other organs in the pelvic area. Symptoms of endometriosis can include painful periods, pelvic pain, and infertility. The exact cause of endometriosis is unknown, but it is thought to be related to hormonal imbalances and genetics. Treatment options for endometriosis may include pain medication, hormone therapy, and surgery to remove the tissue.

SUBCHAPTER 5.3: CHRONIC LYME DISEASE

Chronic Lyme Disease is a controversial condition that some people believe can result from untreated or inadequately treated Lyme Disease. Symptoms of Chronic Lyme Disease can include fatigue, joint pain, and neurological problems. The medical community is divided on whether Chronic Lyme Disease is a real condition, and there is little evidence to suggest that it is caused by a persistent Lyme Disease infection. However, some people with chronic symptoms following Lyme Disease may benefit from treatment for their symptoms.

SUBCHAPTER 5.4: MENIERE'S DISEASE

Meniere's Disease is a disorder of the inner ear that can cause vertigo, hearing loss, and tinnitus (ringing in the ears). The exact cause of Meniere's Disease is unknown, but it is thought to be related to fluid buildup in the inner ear. Treatment options for Meniere's Disease may include medication to relieve symptoms, as well as dietary changes and lifestyle modifications to reduce the risk of vertigo episodes. In this chapter, we have explored some of the lesser-known health conditions that can have a significant impact on a person's life. While these conditions may not be as well-known as others, they are no less important and can benefit from increased awareness and research.

POLYCYSTIC OVARY SYNDROME (PCOS)

Polycystic ovary syndrome (PCOS) is a hormonal disorder that affects women of reproductive age. It is characterized by an excess of male hormones, irregular menstrual cycles, and cysts on the ovaries.

Symptoms

The symptoms of PCOS can vary from woman to woman, and some may experience more severe symptoms than others. Some common symptoms of PCOS include:

- Irregular periods or no periods
- Excess hair growth on the face, chest, stomach, back, or thighs
- Acne
- Weight gain or difficulty losing weight
- Thinning hair or hair loss from the head
- Anxiety or depression

- Difficulty getting pregnant

Treatment

There is currently no cure for PCOS, but it can be managed with proper treatment. Treatment for PCOS may include:

- Birth control pills to regulate menstrual cycles and reduce acne and excess hair growth
- Metformin to improve insulin resistance and regulate blood sugar levels
- Anti-androgen medications to reduce excess hair growth and acne
- Clomiphene (Clomid) to stimulate ovulation and increase the chances of getting pregnant
- Lifestyle changes, such as a healthy diet and exercise, to manage weight and reduce insulin resistance

It is important to work closely with your healthcare provider to develop a treatment plan that is right for you and your specific symptoms. With proper treatment and management, most women with PCOS are able to live healthy, fulfilling lives.

ENDOMETRIOSIS

Endometriosis is a painful condition that affects many women. It occurs when the tissue that usually lines the inside of the uterus grows outside of it, often on the ovaries, fallopian tubes, or tissue lining the pelvis. This displaced tissue responds to the hormonal changes of the menstrual cycle, leading to pain, inflammation, and potentially fertility problems. It is estimated that around 10% of women of reproductive age have endometriosis, but it can take years to diagnose and properly treat. One of the most common symptoms of endometriosis is severe pain during periods, but this can also occur at other times throughout the menstrual cycle. Painful intercourse, chronic pelvic pain, and heavy periods are also common. In some cases, women with endometriosis may experience bowel or urinary problems, tiredness, and infertility. The exact cause of endometriosis is not clear, but there are several theories.

One is that it is caused by retrograde menstruation, where menstrual blood flows back into the pelvis instead of out of the body. Other theories suggest that it is related to genetics or the immune system. There are several treatment options available for endometriosis, depending on the severity of the symptoms and the woman's plans for fertility. Pain relief medication can help manage symptoms, and hormonal treatments such as birth control pills or progestin-only devices can potentially slow the growth of endometrial tissue. In more severe cases, surgery may be necessary to remove the tissue and improve fertility. It is important to talk to a healthcare provider if you experience any symptoms of endometriosis or have concerns about your reproductive health. Early diagnosis and treatment can help manage symptoms and potentially prevent long-term complications.

CHAPTER 5: OTHER LESSER-KNOWN AILMENTS

Subchapter 5.3: Chronic Lyme Disease

Chronic Lyme Disease (CLD) is a complicated illness caused by bacteria transmitted to humans through tick bites. The bacteria that cause Lyme disease are spirochetes, which are spiral-shaped organisms that can enter various tissues and cause a range of symptoms. The disease is transmitted through the bite of an infected tick, and its early symptoms are similar to those of flu. Symptoms of CLD can vary from person to person and can be nonspecific. They can include fatigue, fever, headache, muscle and joint pain, and swollen lymph nodes. CLD can also lead to neurological symptoms, such as brain fog, irritability, memory problems, and depression. Diagnosing CLD can be tricky, as it mimics many other illnesses with similar symptoms. Blood tests can be performed to detect antibodies to Borrelia burgdorferi, the bacteria that causes Lyme disease. However, these tests can give false-negative results, especially in later stages of the disease. Therefore, doctors may rely on clinical diagnosis based on presenting symptoms. The treatment for CLD is a course of antibiotics. The type and length of the antibiotic treatment depend on the stage and severity of the disease. It's crucial to start treatment as soon as possible to prevent the disease from progressing to the chronic stage. In addition to antibiotics, other treatment approaches to CLD include supplements such as vitamins B and D, probiotics, and herbal therapies like garlic and Japanese knotweed. It's also important to support the immune system, boost energy, and improve sleep hygiene. Prevention of tick bites is key in avoiding CLD. Wear protective clothing, check for ticks after being outdoors, and use insect repellent with DEET. Early removal of an attached tick can reduce the risk of transmission of Lyme disease. In conclusion, CLD is a lesser-known ailment that can have severe consequences if left untreated. When caught early, it can be treated with antibiotics. However, prevention is the most effective approach.

CHAPTER 5: OTHER LESSER-KNOWN AILMENTS

Subchapter 5.4: Meniere's Disease

Meniere's Disease is a debilitating disorder that affects the inner ear, leading to hearing loss, tinnitus, vertigo, and often a feeling of pressure or fullness in the ear. It typically affects only one ear, but can sometimes affect both. The exact cause of Meniere's disease is not known, but it is believed to be related to the buildup of fluid in the inner ear. Symptoms of Meniere's disease can be severe and can last for several hours or days. The vertigo can be particularly debilitating and can make it difficult to perform daily activities such as driving or working. While there is no cure for Meniere's disease, there are treatments that can help manage symptoms and improve quality of life. One of the most common treatments for Meniere's disease is a low-salt diet. The excessive buildup of fluid in the inner ear can be exacerbated by a high-salt diet, so reducing salt intake can help reduce symptoms. Other lifestyle changes, such as reducing caffeine and alcohol intake, can also help. Medications such as diuretics can help reduce fluid buildup in the inner ear, while drugs such as anti-nausea medications can help manage symptoms of vertigo and nausea. In some cases, injections of steroids or other medications directly into the inner ear can also help reduce symptoms. Surgical options may be considered in severe cases of Meniere's disease that do not respond to other treatments. One common surgical procedure is a procedure called endolymphatic sac decompression, which involves surgery on the inner ear to reduce fluid buildup. If you are experiencing symptoms of Meniere's disease, it is important to consult with a healthcare provider. Early diagnosis and treatment can help manage symptoms and improve quality of life.

Hidden Health Conditions: Understanding and Treating Lesser-Known Ailments

CHAPTER 6: TREATMENT OPTIONS FOR HIDDEN HEALTH CONDITIONS

Hidden health conditions can be challenging to diagnose and manage due to their complex nature. Treatment options vary depending on the condition and individual needs. In this chapter, we will explore traditional medical treatments, alternative and complementary therapies, as well as lifestyle changes for long-term management.

Traditional Medical Treatments

Traditional medical treatments for hidden health conditions typically involve medications and therapies prescribed by a healthcare provider. In some cases, surgical intervention may be necessary. For digestive conditions such as celiac disease or SIBO, a gluten-free diet or antibiotics may be prescribed, respectively. In the case of nerve-related conditions such as fibromyalgia or migraines, pain medications or anti-inflammatory drugs may be prescribed. Immune system conditions such as lupus or rheumatoid arthritis may require immunosuppressant medications to manage symptoms and prevent flare-ups. It is important to communicate regularly with your healthcare provider to evaluate the effectiveness of your treatment plan and make adjustments as needed.

Alternative and Complementary Therapies

Alternative and complementary therapies offer a holistic approach to managing hidden health conditions. These therapies can be used in conjunction with traditional medical treatments or as standalone therapies. Acupuncture has been shown to be effective in managing chronic pain conditions such as fibromyalgia. Massage therapy and chiropractic adjustments can help alleviate tension and pain associated with nerve-related conditions. Herbal remedies and dietary supplements may also be used as part of a holistic treatment plan. It is essential to consult with a qualified practitioner before pursuing alternative or complementary therapies, as some remedies may interact with medications or exacerbate symptoms.

Lifestyle Changes for Long-Term Management

Lifestyle changes can support long-term management of hidden health conditions. Maintaining a healthy diet and regular exercise routine can improve digestive and immune system health, as well as help manage chronic pain conditions. Reducing stress through meditation, mindfulness practices, or therapy can help alleviate symptoms associated with nerve-related conditions. Regular sleep habits and relaxation exercises can also support overall health and well-being. In some cases, environmental factors may prolong or trigger hidden health condition symptoms. Identifying and avoiding triggers such as allergens or pollutants may also be an important part of long-term management. Overall, a combination of traditional medical treatments, alternative and complementary therapies, and lifestyle changes can empower individuals to manage and improve their hidden health conditions. Working closely with healthcare providers and qualified practitioners can help individuals create a comprehensive treatment plan tailored to their individual needs.

TRADITIONAL MEDICAL TREATMENTS

When it comes to treating hidden health conditions, traditional medical treatments are some of the most common methods used by healthcare professionals. While some of these treatments may not always be effective for everyone, they have been shown to improve the symptoms of many lesser-known ailments. One of the most widespread traditional medical treatments is medication. For instance, those with fibromyalgia or chronic fatigue syndrome may use antidepressants or anti-seizure drugs to help manage their symptoms. Similarly, people with migraines may use medications ranging from over-the-counter painkillers to prescription migraine-specific medications to prevent and alleviate attacks. Other treatments may include surgeries or procedures. For individuals with endometriosis, laparoscopic surgery to remove lesions or hysterectomy may be necessary to reduce symptoms. For those with gastroparesis, a gastric pacemaker or botulinum toxin injections may be used to stimulate stomach contractions and improve digestion. It's worth noting that traditional treatments are often accompanied by side effects and may not work for everyone. It's important to work with a healthcare professional to determine the best course of treatment for one's specific condition and lifestyle. Overall, traditional medical treatments remain a common and important part of managing hidden health conditions and improving quality of life for those who live with them.

ALTERNATIVE AND COMPLEMENTARY THERAPIES

While traditional medical treatments are often the primary choice for those with hidden health conditions, alternative and complementary therapies can also play a significant role in managing symptoms and improving overall well-being. One popular alternative therapy is acupuncture, which involves the insertion of thin needles into specific points on the body. It has been found to be effective in treating chronic pain, fibromyalgia, and migraines. Another increasingly popular therapy is chiropractic care, which focuses on the manipulation of the spine to improve overall health and alleviate pain. It has been found to be helpful in treating a variety of conditions, including back pain and migraines. Massage therapy is another complementary therapy that has been found to be beneficial for those with hidden health conditions, including fibromyalgia and chronic fatigue syndrome. It can help to reduce muscle tension and promote relaxation, leading to a reduction in symptoms. Herbal supplements and nutritional therapy are also commonly used complementary therapies for managing hidden health conditions. Supplements such as fish oil and magnesium have been found to be effective in reducing inflammation and alleviating pain, while nutritional therapy can help to support overall health and address specific deficiencies. It's important to note that while alternative and complementary therapies can be effective, it's essential to consult with a healthcare professional before starting any new treatment. They can provide guidance on which therapies may be most beneficial for your individual needs and help ensure that any therapy you choose is safe and effective.

SUBCHAPTER 6.3: LIFESTYLE CHANGES FOR LONG-TERM MANAGEMENT

In order to manage hidden health conditions over the long-term, it is often necessary to make significant lifestyle changes. While medical treatments and therapies can certainly help manage symptoms, adopting healthy habits and making positive changes to your daily routine can have a significant impact on your overall health and wellness. One of the most important lifestyle changes you can make is to adopt a healthy diet. For many hidden health conditions, what you eat can have a major impact on your symptoms. For example, people with celiac disease need to avoid gluten, while those with SIBO may need to limit their intake of certain types of carbohydrates. Eating a balanced diet that is rich in fruits, vegetables, lean protein, and healthy fats can also help keep your body functioning optimally. Exercise is another important lifestyle change that can help manage hidden health conditions. Regular physical activity can help improve muscle strength, boost energy levels, and promote better sleep quality. If you have a condition that makes it difficult to exercise, such as fibromyalgia or chronic fatigue syndrome, it may be helpful to work with a physical therapist to develop a safe and effective exercise plan. Managing stress is another important factor in managing hidden health conditions. Stress can trigger symptoms and exacerbate existing conditions, so finding ways to reduce stress in your daily life is crucial. This might include practicing relaxation techniques such as deep breathing or meditation, or finding enjoyable activities that help you unwind, such as yoga or spending time in nature. Finally, it is important to get plenty of restful sleep. For many hidden health conditions, poor sleep quality and insomnia are common symptoms. Developing good sleep hygiene habits, such as avoiding screens before bed and creating a calming sleep environment, can help improve sleep quality and promote better overall health. By making these lifestyle changes and adopting healthy habits, you can help manage hidden health conditions and enjoy better quality of life over the long-term. While it may take time to establish new habits, the benefits of a healthy lifestyle are well worth the effort.

Conclusion

The world of hidden health conditions is vast and complex, impacting millions of people worldwide. From digestive problems to immune system disorders and beyond, these often-overlooked ailments can significantly affect a person's quality of life. Despite this, many lesser-known conditions are still misunderstood by the general public and even medical professionals. In this book, we have explored some of the most common hidden health conditions, including celiac disease, lupus, and chronic fatigue syndrome. We have also looked at treatment options, including traditional medical treatments, alternative and complementary therapies, and lifestyle changes. It is our hope that this book has shed light on these lesser-known ailments and empowered readers to seek the proper diagnosis and treatment they deserve. By raising awareness and increasing understanding, we can work towards a world where hidden health conditions are recognized and treated with the same urgency and respect as more widely understood illnesses. If you suspect you may be suffering from a hidden health condition, we encourage you to seek the advice of a medical professional. With the proper diagnosis and treatment, you can take control of your health and find relief from even the most elusive and complex of ailments.

RECAP OF HIDDEN HEALTH CONDITIONS

Throughout this book, we have discussed a variety of hidden health conditions that impact people every day. We've highlighted how these ailments can affect people's lives, both physically and emotionally, and shared some of the most common symptoms associated with each condition. Some of the most common ailments we've covered include celiac disease, gastroparesis, fibromyalgia, lupus, and chronic fatigue syndrome. We've explored their causes and looked at both traditional and alternative treatment options.

CALL TO ACTION FOR BETTER RECOGNITION AND TREATMENT

While great strides have been made in recent years to raise awareness of many of these conditions, there is still much work to be done. It is essential that we continue to advocate for greater recognition and support for individuals dealing with hidden health conditions. We must work to educate not only the general public but also medical professionals on the importance of recognizing and treating these lesser-known ailments properly. With greater understanding and better tools at our disposal, we can improve outcomes for millions of people around the world.

FINAL THOUGHTS AND RESOURCES

We hope that the information provided in this book has been helpful to you. Remember that you are not alone in your struggles with hidden health conditions, and help is available. Don't be afraid to reach out to your healthcare provider or a support group for assistance. Here are some resources to aid you in your journey towards better health: - The National Institute of Neurological Disorders and Stroke - The American Autoimmune Related Diseases Association - National Organization for Rare Disorders - The Ehlers-Danlos Society - Chronic Illness Support Groups Remember that knowledge is power, and with the right tools and resources at your disposal, you can take steps towards better health and a more fulfilling life.

SUBCHAPTER 7.1: RECAP OF HIDDEN HEALTH CONDITIONS

Throughout this book, we have explored various Hidden Health Conditions - ailments that are not commonly talked about or recognized despite affecting a significant population. In Chapter 2, we discussed conditions related to the Digestive System, including Celiac Disease, Gastroparesis, Small Intestinal Bacterial Overgrowth (SIBO), and Irritable Bowel Syndrome (IBS). These conditions can cause discomfort and affect one's daily life if not properly managed. Chapter 3 went on to explore the Nervous System and its related conditions such as Fibromyalgia, Chronic Fatigue Syndrome, Restless Leg Syndrome, and Migraines. These conditions can be debilitating and severely impact one's quality of life. Chapter 4 focused on the Immune System and its associated conditions such as Lupus, Multiple Sclerosis (MS), Sjogren's Syndrome, and Rheumatoid Arthritis (RA). These conditions can have a significant impact on one's health and may require vigilant management. Chapter 5 delved into Other Lesser-Known Ailments, such as Polycystic Ovary Syndrome (PCOS), Endometriosis, Chronic Lyme Disease, and Meniere's Disease. These conditions, although not as widely recognized, can have a significant impact on one's well-being. Lastly, Chapter 6 explored various Treatment Options for Hidden Health Conditions, including both traditional medical treatments and alternative and complementary therapies. Lifestyle changes were also highlighted as effective ways to manage and cope with these conditions in the long term. Overall, the main purpose of this book is to shed light on these Hidden Health Conditions and provide valuable information to those affected by them. It is our hope that this book will help improve recognition and treatment of these lesser-known ailments, ultimately leading to improved quality of life for those who suffer from them.

CALL TO ACTION FOR BETTER RECOGNITION AND TREATMENT

Hidden health conditions can be incredibly challenging to live with. For years, patients with these conditions have been misdiagnosed, mistreated, or simply ignored, leaving them feeling isolated and helpless. However, there is hope for better recognition and treatment of these ailments. The first step in improving recognition and treatment for hidden health conditions is to raise awareness. Many patients suffer for years before they receive accurate diagnoses. By increasing public awareness of these conditions, more people can recognize their symptoms and seek proper medical care. Secondly, there need to be more specialized medical professionals trained to recognize and treat these conditions. Medical schools and training programs should include more extensive training on the less common illnesses covered in this book to prepare professionals for diagnosing and treating hidden health conditions. Thirdly, there need to be more resources and funding devoted to research and development of treatments for these ailments. Studies on the pathophysiology of these conditions, as well as clinical trials for new treatments, should be conducted with more funding in order to provide better treatment options for patients. Fourthly, patients with hidden health conditions need to advocate for themselves and demand better care. This can be done by speaking up about their experiences, seeking out medical professionals who specialize in their conditions, and seeking out support groups for their specific condition. Lastly, insurance companies and healthcare systems need to recognize and support patients with hidden health conditions. These ailments often require extensive medical care, which can be costly.

Insurance companies and healthcare systems should provide coverage for patients with these conditions to ensure that they receive the necessary care. By raising awareness, training medical professionals, funding research and development, supporting patients, and recognizing the need for appropriate coverage, we can improve recognition and treatment of hidden health conditions. With these steps, we can work towards improving the lives of millions of individuals living with these lesser-known ailments.

Final Thoughts and Resources

In conclusion, Hidden Health Conditions: Understanding and Treating Lesser-Known Ailments sheds light on a variety of conditions that are often overlooked. The purpose of this book is to provide information on these conditions that can help patients and their loved ones understand their illnesses and find the best treatment options available. Remember, if you or someone you know may be suffering from a hidden health condition, there is hope for better recognition and treatment. It is important to advocate for yourself or your loved one, seek out specialized medical professionals, and never give up hope for a better tomorrow. Here are some additional resources for individuals seeking more information on hidden health conditions: - National Organization for Rare Disorders (NORD) - The Ehlers-Danlos Society - Dysautonomia International - International Foundation for Gastrointestinal Disorders - National Institute of Mental Health - The American Autoimmune Related Diseases Association (AARDA)